I0697453

NOVICE KEGEL EXERCISES

Ultimate Guide To Complete Kegel Fitness Manual For Beginners

FRANK BOBBY

Copyright © 2023 By Frank Bobby,

Please note that you must obtain explicit written consent from the publisher before reproducing, disseminating, or transmitting any part of this publication.

This applies to all methods, including photocopying, recording, or any other electronic or mechanical means. It's important to note that short excerpts that are smoothly integrated into reviews and noncommercial applications allowed by copyright law might not be subject to this restriction.

All Rights Reserved.

Table of Contents

Introductory

Kegel exercises, also known as pelvic floor exercises, are regimens designed to strengthen the pelvic floor muscles.

The pelvic floor muscles are essential for sustaining urinary and bowel continence as they support the pelvic organs. Urinary incontinence (the involuntary loss of bladder control) or pelvic organ prolapse can result from weakened pelvic floor muscles due to pregnancy, childbirth, aging, obesity, or certain medical conditions.

By repeatedly contracting and relaxing the pelvic floor muscles, Kegel exercises seek to strengthen and tone these muscles. Both genders can benefit from these exercises. Here is a comprehensive guide to performing Kegel exercises:

• To strengthen your pelvic floor, the first stage is to identify the appropriate muscles. Women may attempt midstream urination while seated on the commode. The muscles of your pelvic floor are responsible for this action. Males can attempt to contract the muscles responsible for defecation.

- It is recommended that the bladder be emptied prior to commencing the exercises to prevent any discomfort or disruptions.

- After locating the pelvic floor muscles, they should be contracted by squeezing and lifting them upward. Consider the difficulty of restraining a gastrointestinal movement or preventing flatulence. Instead of tensing your abdominal, quadriceps, and buttock muscles, relax them.

- Maintain the contraction: Beginning with a squeeze duration of approximately 5 seconds, gradually increase it to 10 seconds as your muscles become stronger.

• After each set of contractions, release the muscles for approximately 10 seconds.

• Exercise by cycling through ten repetitions of contractions followed by relaxations. Attempt to exercise at least three times per day.

When conducting Kegel exercises, it is essential to breathe normally and avoid holding your breath or straining. They are adaptable enough to be performed seated, standing, or reclining down. Consistency and regularity are essential because significant changes can take weeks or even months to manifest.

If you have urinary incontinence or other pelvic floor-related issues, you should consult with a physician or physical therapist who specializes in pelvic floor rehabilitation. You can receive advice and recommendations tailored to your specific situation.

CHAPTER ONE
Benefits Of Performing Kegel Exercises

There are many benefits to performing Kegel exercises, and not just for women. Among the principal advantages are the following:

• Strengthening the pelvic floor muscles is the primary advantage of performing Kegel exercises. The regular use and exercise of these muscles can increase their strength and endurance. You can avoid pelvic organ prolapse and have improved bladder and bowel control by doing so.

• Kegel exercises are frequently recommended as a non-invasive method of treating urinary incontinence. Coughing, sneezing, chuckling, and exercise are among the activities that can cause urine leakage.

• It is common for the pelvic floor muscles to weaken following childbirth. Kegel exercises are extremely beneficial for postpartum recovery and muscle conditioning. This can aid recovery from an episiotomy or perineal injury and reduce the likelihood of postpartum urinary incontinence.

- Training and sustaining strong pelvic floor muscles may lead to improvements in sexual health and satisfaction. It has been demonstrated that Kegel exercises enhance arousal, orgasmic strength, and vaginal tightness by increasing blood flow to the pelvic region and enhancing muscular tone.

- Pregnant women are advised to perform Kegel exercises to prepare their pelvic floor muscles for the physical demands of labor and delivery. By strengthening these muscles, pushing during labor can be made simpler and complications such as tears and damage can be avoided.

• Kegel exercises are beneficial for men because they strengthen the pelvic floor muscles, including those that support the prostate organ. Regular Kegel exercises may result in a healthier prostate, improved urinary control, and fewer symptoms of BPH.

Keep in mind that results may differ from person to person, and that performing Kegel exercises correctly and consistently is crucial for their success. If you have specific questions or concerns about your pelvic floor, it's best to consult a specialist, who can provide you with individualized guidance.

When Are Kegel Exercises Beneficial?

Many individuals, not just women, can strengthen their pelvic floor muscles and improve their pelvic health by performing Kegel exercises. Below are some examples of individuals who would benefit from performing Kegel exercises:

• Kegel exercises are frequently prescribed for women with urinary incontinence, including stress incontinence (urinary leakage during activities such as coughing, sneezing, or exercising) and urge incontinence (involuntary leakage due to sudden and intense urges to urinate).

• Due to a weakening of the pelvic floor muscles, urinary incontinence and pelvic organ prolapse are two conditions that can affect women during and after pregnancy. Performing Kegel exercises during pregnancy and after childbirth has numerous advantages, including enhanced urinary control and accelerated recovery.

• Kegel exercises can assist men with urinary incontinence, whether it's due to a hyperactive bladder, a history of prostate surgery, or another cause. Strengthening the pelvic floor muscles may lead to enhanced bladder control and fewer accidents.

• Prolapse is the condition that occurs when pelvic organs such as the bladder, uterus, or rectum descend and impinge on the vaginal walls. Kegel exercises, which strengthen and support the pelvic floor, may alleviate symptoms and prevent future prolapse if performed regularly.

• Those with fecal incontinence (the involuntary loss of bowel control) may find relief by performing Kegel exercises. The ability to control bowel movements and reduce the frequency of leakage can be enhanced by strengthening the pelvic floor muscles.

• Kegel exercises may not be an effective treatment for erectile dysfunction (ED) on their own, but they can improve the overall sexual health of males. Kegel exercises, which concentrate on strengthening the pelvic floor muscles, may improve erectile function and increase blood flow to the pelvic region.

• Athletes and other physically active individuals: Kegel exercises can prevent injury in high-impact sports such as boxing and mixed martial arts. If you want your core muscles to provide more support and stability during exercise, you should focus on strengthening your pelvic floor muscles.

Before beginning Kegel exercises, it is best to consult with a doctor or physical therapist who specializes in pelvic floor rehabilitation for specific recommendations tailored to your requirements.

CHAPTER TWO
The Pelvic Floor: Essential Information

The pelvic floor's muscles, ligaments, and connective tissues form a sling-like support system for the pelvis. Due to this structure, the rectum, bladder, and uterus (in females) all find stable footing.

To gain a deeper understanding of the pelvic floor, contemplate the following:

1. Anatomically, the pelvic floor is composed of a group of muscles that stabilize and direct the pelvic organs. These muscles include the iliococcygeus (IC), puborectalis (PR), and pubococcygeus (PC).

2. The pelvic floor is situated between the pubis and the coccyx. It extends between the two sets of ischial tuberosities.

3. The pelvic floor muscles have multiple functions, including but not limited to the following:

• By providing support, they maintain the pelvic organs in their proper positions and prevent prolapse (when they fall into the rectus or vaginal canal).

• The pelvic floor muscles are crucial for preserving the ability to regulate urination and defecation. By governing the anus and urethra, they help to regulate urination.

• Sexual function: These muscles help men maintain an erection, women maintain vaginal tone and elasticity, and both sexes have satisfying orgasms.

• Stability: The pelvic floor muscles, along with the deep abdominal and back muscles, support the core and contribute to the maintenance of correct posture.

4. Some of the symptoms that can result from weak or dysfunctional pelvic floor muscles include urinary incontinence, fecal incontinence, pelvic organ prolapse, erectile dysfunction, and low back pain. The causes of pelvic floor dysfunction include, but are not limited to, pregnancy, childbirth, aging, obesity, hormonal changes, persistent wheezing, and certain medical conditions.

5. Kegel exercises, which target the pelvic floor muscles, are frequently prescribed to improve pelvic floor strength and function, emphasizing their significance.

By contracting and relaxing the pelvic floor muscles, these exercises aim to strengthen them.

Strengthening the pelvic floor can aid in the treatment of incontinence, provide support for the pelvic organs, and lessen other associated issues.

Those who understand the importance of the pelvic floor are better equipped to care for it and deal with any potential problems.

Consult a urologist, gynecologist, or physical therapist who specializes in pelvic floor health if you are experiencing issues with or have concerns about your pelvic floor.

How To Preparation For Kegels

Before commencing Kegel exercises, it is essential to take a few basic precautions to prevent injury. As preparation aids, here are some suggestions:

• Become familiar with the proper form for performing Kegel exercises. Learn when to use which pelvic floor muscles and how to contract and release them. Please review the earlier portions of this conversation for a detailed explanation of how to proceed.

• Choose a private, tranquil location where you will not be interrupted while performing Kegel exercises. This may help you become more attuned to the movements and sensations of the pelvic floor.

• Before commencing Kegel exercises, make sure your bladder is empty. A full bladder may impede the normal contraction and relaxation of the pelvic floor muscles.

• Deep breathing can help you relax and maintain proper form while exercising. Take a few deep breaths before beginning, and strive to maintain calm and regular breathing throughout the workout.

• Establish a routine: Consistency is required to see results from Kegel exercises. Create a workout schedule, whether you exercise daily or a few times per week. Schedule your exercises in advance to ensure they remain a regular part of your routine.

• Those unfamiliar with Kegel exercises or with a weak pelvic floor should begin cautiously. As your muscles adapt, begin with fewer repetitions and shorter contractions and gradually increase to maximum intensity. Initial overuse of muscles can result in discomfort or fatigue.

• The effects of Kegel exercises, like those of any other fitness regimen, may not be immediately apparent. Practice with perseverance and diligence. The strength and function of the pelvic floor may not improve until several weeks or months of consistent exercise.

• If you have specific concerns or issues regarding your pelvic floor, it may be advisable to consult a medical professional. A specialist in pelvic floor rehabilitation, such as a physician or physical therapist, can provide you with specific instructions, an evaluation of your technique, and individualized recommendations.

You can maximize the benefits of Kegel exercises and improve the health of your pelvic floor if you perform them frequently and give yourself ample time to prepare. Always pay attention to your body and consult a physician if you have any questions or concerns.

CHAPTER THREE
Starting Kegels

In fundamental Kegel exercises, the pelvic floor muscles are exercised and relaxed. Here is a comprehensive breakdown of the basic Kegel exercises:

• Pay close attention to the region between your anus and vagina or scrotum; this is where your pelvic floor muscles are located. You can attempt to urinate in a trickle by retaining your bladder until the flow of urine ceases. Only when absolutely necessary, such as during the identification procedure, should this be done.

• Assume a comfortable position; Kegel exercises can be performed while seated, reclining down, or standing. Choose a seat where you will feel most comfortable.

• Before beginning the exercises, take several steady breaths to calm your mind and body. It is essential to maintain a calm demeanor throughout the exercises.

• Squeeze and raise the pelvic floor muscles as if you were attempting to prevent urination or gas release. Only contract the muscles of your pelvic floor; do not tense your abdomen, buttocks, or thighs.

• Do not release your muscle groups for a few seconds after contracting them. Beginning with a 3- to 5-second hold, gradually increase the time to 10 seconds as your muscles become stronger. Don't neglect to maintain normal breathing even when holding.

• It is essential to completely release the pelvic floor muscles for the same amount of time that they were contracted. There should be a brief inter-set interlude.

• The objective of this exercise is to complete ten consecutive sets of contractions and relaxations, which you should repeat. The preceding set of Kegel exercises constitutes one cycle.

You can progressively increase the number of rounds you perform as you adjust to the routine and gain strength.

• Maintain a regular schedule, ideally performing three Kegel exercises daily. If you desire the finest results, consistency is essential.

It is possible for the strength and endurance of the pelvic floor to vary between individuals. The duration and intensity of your exercises should be gradually increased over time.

Consult a physician or physical therapist if you are experiencing discomfort or other health issues. They can offer individualized guidance.

The Advancement Of Kegels

To strengthen the pelvic floor muscles, more challenging variations of the conventional Kegel exercises are performed. Once you've mastered the basics, you may want to incorporate some of the more advanced moves listed below.

• Rapid muscle contractions: swiftly and forcefully contract your pelvic floor muscles. The muscles should be contracted as quickly and as firmly as possible, and then released. Create a rippling or pulsing motion by contracting and relaxing your muscles rapidly. The suggested initial number of repetitions is ten.

• Put yourself to the test by holding the contraction for an extended duration than usual. Increase its duration until it lasts at least 20 seconds. Using this technique, the strength of the muscles supporting the pelvic floor can be increased.

• Perform progressive contractions, in which you contract your muscles progressively. Start with a mild contraction, gradually increase the intensity to a moderate level, and then gradually release the contraction. This method simulates the physical sensation of bladder or intestinal pressure gradually rising and declining.

• You can simultaneously strengthen your pelvic floor and other muscles by performing combination exercises.

Lifting one leg off the floor or performing a crunch while simultaneously engaging the pelvic floor muscles are two excellent examples. Combined motions utilize more muscles and test the coordination and stamina of the pelvic floor.

• Strengthen your pelvic floor muscles with resistance training by performing Kegel exercises with weighted spheres or other devices. This resistance can enhance the difficulty of muscle-building exercises.

• Coordinate your breathing with the contractions and relaxations of your pelvic floor muscles (a more advanced breathing technique). Inhale deeply, and as you exhale, contract and raise your muscles. When taking a deep inhalation, you should relax and let go.

Enhanced mind-muscle coordination and general control of the pelvic floor can be attained through coordinated respiration.

It is essential to give attention to your body and move at a pace that feels natural to you. If you are experiencing pain, discomfort, or concerns, consults a doctor or physical therapist specializing in pelvic floor rehabilitation.

They will be able to provide you with individualized instructions

and monitor your form to ensure
that you are performing the
complex movements safely.

CHAPTER FOUR
Including Resistance Exercise

Add resistance training to your Kegel regimen if you want to strengthen and tone your pelvic floor muscles even further. Here are some suggestions for getting started with resistance training:

1. Kegel spheres or weighted vaginal cones are devices intended to be inserted into the vagina and used to make Kegel exercises more challenging.

As your pelvic floor muscles become stronger, you can modify the resistance of these tools by selecting a heavier or larger device.

You should start with a lighter weight and gradually increase to a heavier one.

• Kegel spheres or weights are inserted into the vagina while the user contracts her pelvic floor muscles to maintain their position.

Perform Kegel exercises with a focus on contracting and elevating the muscles while maintaining the apparatus in position. It is recommended to gradually hold the device for longer and longer durations.

2. Resistance bands (elastic bands) offer some form of resistance when extended. Consider utilizing a resistance band to intensify your Kegel exercises. How? Keep reading!

• Place your feet level on the floor or perch on the chair's edge.

• Wrap the resistance band around the upper quadriceps, just above the knees.

• To perform Kegels, contract and elevate the pelvic floor muscles against the resistance of the band.

• Contract for the desired amount of time, and then terminate.

• Continue in this manner until you've completed the specified number of sets.

• When utilizing a resistance band, ensure that it is not too taut so that you can exercise with proper form and a complete range of motion.

3. Using your palms as resistance during Kegel exercises is an additional method for intensifying your workout.

You can exercise the pelvic floor muscles by applying mild finger pressure and lifting the sagging skin. Place your fingertips within the vagina (for women) or between the scrotum and anus (for men) to contract your pelvic floor muscles.

Remember that you should commence with a lower level of resistance and gradually increase it. While exercising, you should never exceed the point of physical discomfort or agony.

If you are interested in beginning a resistance training program, it is best to consult a physician or pelvic floor physical therapist who can advise you on the best exercises, equipment, and schedule.

They will be able to provide you with specific guidance and monitor your form to ensure that you maximize your workout.

How Frequently And For How Long Should You Perform Kegel Exercises?

Your needs and objectives will determine the frequency and duration of your Kegel exercises. Consider the following advice if you're having difficulty establishing a regimen.

How frequently:

• Kegel exercises should be performed at least three times per day to begin.

- Spread out your exercises throughout the day if you want to give your muscles a rest.

• You can increase the number of times per day to as many as four or five as you acquire confidence and experience.

The duration:

Start by holding each contraction for three to five seconds, then releasing it.

• You should progressively increase the duration of your workouts as your muscles become stronger and more accustomed to them. Aim to hold each contraction for at least 10 seconds.

• In a similar manner, increase the number of repetitions or sets with each workout. Beginning with 10 repetitions, progressively increase to 20.

Pay close attention to your body and recover when it prompts you to do so. Reduce the difficulty or duration of your workouts and consult a physician if you continue to experience pain or discomfort during or after your workouts.

Performing Kegel exercises on a regular basis is essential. Exercising for a lengthy period of time at once is less beneficial than exercising consistently for a shorter period of time. A series of shorter, more intense exercises throughout the day are preferable to a single marathon session.

A physician or physical therapist who specializes in pelvic floor health can provide you with individualized advice and recommendations based on your specific requirements and concerns.

CHAPTER FIVE
Resolution Of Obstacles And Progress

To ensure that you are performing Kegel exercises correctly and maximizing their benefits, you should focus on troubleshooting and progression. If you are experiencing difficulties with Kegel exercises, here are some solutions:

1. Having difficulty identifying the correct muscles:

• If you cannot locate your pelvic floor muscles when evacuating, try the "stop and start" method. Only when absolutely necessary, such as during the identification procedure, should this be done.

• Another option is to insert a clean finger into the vagina (for women) or the area between the scrotum and the anus (for men) and contract the surrounding muscles. Light pressure should be experienced.

2. Uncoupling from sensation and/or muscle:

• Try a different position if you cannot feel your muscles tightening or if they feel limp. Try seated, standing, and lying down to determine the most effective muscle-engaging posture.

- Focus more on the effectiveness of the contraction than on its magnitude. Ensure that you are only contracting the pelvic floor muscles and not your abdominal or buttock muscles as well.

- Visualize the muscles contracting and tightening, or the passage of urine or gas being obstructed.

3. Constriction or constriction of the diaphragm:

- Maintain slow, relaxed respiration while performing Kegel exercises. Avoid contracting your pelvic floor muscles by not inhaling deeply or by exerting yourself excessively.

• Relax and tense your muscles as you go through the motions by taking slow, deep breathing. synchronize your respiration and muscle contractions.

4. Stopping or reducing speed:

• If you feel that your progress has plateaued, it may be time to increase the difficulty of your exercise regimen. Either increase the time between repetitions or the number of sets you perform to further challenge your musculature.

• Quick contractions, sustained contractions, and strength training with Kegel balls and resistance bands are all practices classified as "advanced." These adjustments can be a welcome change of pace that propels you forward.

• Have your pelvic floor strength and function regularly assessed by a medical specialist. They can evaluate your current fitness level, monitor your progress, and recommend necessary adjustments to your regimen.

5. Consult a physician for advice:

• Kegel exercises are beneficial, but if you're having difficulty getting started or have specific questions or concerns, it's best to consult a doctor or a pelvic floor physical therapist. They may evaluate your technique, offer customized guidance, and assist you in resolving any underlying issues that are impeding your development.

Maintain your Kegel exercises with perseverance and consistency. Improving the strength and function of the pelvic floor can take time, and consistent practice is required to see results.

The Conclusion

Kegel exercises are an effective means of strengthening and maintaining the pelvic floor. Regular practice of these exercises has been shown to improve bladder control, strengthen pelvic organs, heighten sexual delight, and enhance pelvic floor health as a whole.

The benefits of Kegel exercises are maximized when the proper technique is employed, adequate preparation is made, and a regular schedule is adhered to. Beginning with basic contractions and progressing to more advanced variations, incorporating weight training if desired, and resolving any potential obstacles will yield optimal results.

Pay attention to your body, make the necessary adjustments, and consult a medical professional if you have persistent or specific concerns or issues. They can tailor their instructions to your particular aims and objectives, review your form, and offer additional suggestions.

Persistence and consistency are essential. You will appreciate the numerous benefits of robust pelvic floor muscles if you make Kegel exercises a regular part of your routine and maintain your commitment to pelvic floor health.

THE END

57

www.ingramcontent.com/pod-product-compliance
Lightning Source LLC
Chambersburg PA
CBHW060808260726
48660CB00002B/843